Summer, Sleep & Repeat

Science-Backed Strategies to Sleep Better, Beat Insomnia and Rest on Hot Days and Nights

Dr. Fredy A. Escobar Ipuz

Copyright © 2020 Fredy A. Escobar Ipuz
All rights reserved.
ISBN: 9798665323312

Dedication

Dedicated to my patients, in your deep and restful sleep lies unlimited power.

Especially for my family, a living example of love and unconditional support.

Table Of Contents

Prologue i
Introduction ii
Global Warming iv
Chapter 1: Normal Sleep: A Comprehensive Background 1
  1.1 Wakefulness 3
  1.2 Sleep 5
      Non-REM (NREM) Sleep 7
      REM sleep 9
  1.3 Sleep Mechanisms (the two process-model) 11
      Process S (Homeostatic system) 12
      Process C (Circadian system) 15

Chapter 2: Challenges To Sleep In Summer Or Hot Weather 21
  2.1 Seasonal Effects on Sleep 22
  2.2 Summer Sleep Disruptors 23
      Long Days 23
      Hot Nights (the temperature effect) 24
      Vacation Jet Lag 25
      Too Much Alcohol 25
      Spicy Foods 26
      Afternoon Naps 26
      Mosquitoes and Other Bugs 27
      Allergies 27
      Lack of Deep Sleep 28

Lack of Exercise 28

Poor Sleep Hygiene 29

Poor Air Quality and Humidity in Our Room 29

Chapter 3: Evidence-Based Recommendations For Summer Sleep 32

3.1 Don't Neglect Your Sleep Schedule 33

    Your Wake-Up Time 34

    Your Sleep Time 35

3.2 Control Light Source Exposure 35

3.3 Regulate Your Internal Temperature 38

3.4 Choose Natural Fibers 39

3.5 Trick Your Sheets 40

3.6 Use a Cold Water Bottle 40

3.7 Keep Your Feet and Hands Out 40

3.8 Check Your Sleepwear 41

3.9 Wet Your Pulses 41

3.10 Soak Your Feet 41

3.11 Use a Flannel 41

3.12 Use a Rice sock, Thermic Seed Bags or Gel Packs 42

3.13 Mist a Cooling Spray 42

3.14 Use a Fan 42

3.15 Ice the Air 43

3.16 Refrain from Cold Showers 43

3.17 Improve the Thermal Conditions and Indoor Air Quality (IAQ). 44

3.18 Open the Doors and Windows 45

3.19 Ventilate the Attic 45

3.20 Move Rooms 45

3.21 Keep the Stove Off 46

3.22 Use a Dehumidifier 46

3.23 Get Outside 46

Chapter 4: Other Related Tips 48

4.1 Check Your Diet 49

4.2 Stay Hydrated 51

4.3 Limit Social Interactions in the Evening 52

4.4 Exercise 53

4.5 Hang Clothes Outside 54

4.6 Clean Your Gutters 54

4.7 Sleep in a Hammock 54

4.8 Use Cooling/Migraine Patches 55

4.9 Never Forget Your Medication 55

4.10 Try a Wool Mattress Topper 55

4.11 Unplug Your Electronics 56

4.12 Invest in Desiccants 56

4.13 Listen to the Rain 56

4.14 Try Pranayama 57

4.15 Maintain Proper Sleep Hygiene 57

Conclusion 60
References 61
About the Author 67

PROLOGUE

I was born and grew up in a city that not only stands out for the immense warmth of its citizens, but also for its high temperatures throughout the year. Life has offered me the opportunity to visit other regions of the world, where the high temperatures too, especially in summer, are not a friendly sleeping partner. I know what it is really like to sleep in the summer season or in regions with climates that only offer high temperatures all year round.

Sleep is essential, and for quite a long time, year after year, especially in summer, patients call me complaining of sleep problems and asking for recommendations on how to get better sleep. Summer is not a bad time to sleep, as it is the best time of the year for sleep restoration. It is the best season to free ourselves from the burden of accumulated sleep deprivation due to work stress, academic responsibilities, and household duties.

For this reason, I have compiled a series of explanations and recommendations based on scientific literature, that can serve as a guide to help you sleep better, and survive the warm summer nights or places that are known for having high temperatures.

Yes, in summer it's possible to get a good night's sleep without problems.

INTRODUCTION

Do you often wonder why you have a hard time getting enough sleep during summer, despite doing several things you otherwise thought would bring about restful sleep?

Are you also looking for a guide that will enlighten you on the inner workings of sleep, and how you can use that knowledge to sleep better during summer and every other season, all year round?

If you've answered YES, keep reading...

You are about to discover the inner workings of sleep as well as how to optimize your sleep during summer!

Every year as summer approaches, a lot of people have plans of going on vacation, sunning on the beach, trying out a variety of summer drinks, resting up and catching up on sleep.

Unfortunately, every year, a lot of these people end up disappointed when things don't turn out as they envisioned. Instead of being rested, they find themselves wishing they had a vacation to recover from their vacation.

Perhaps the reason you are here is because you've experienced the same or have noticed a pattern of not being well-rested during summer, and are looking for answers to all the questions running through your mind...

Why is it that I'm having a hard time falling asleep and staying asleep?

Why don't I feel well-rested whenever I wake up?

Why do I feel fatigued, tired and without energy during the day?

What is it I am doing wrong?

How can I turn things around?

What do I need to do, and what do I need to stop doing?

What does science say about sleep and summer?

If you have these and other related questions, this book is for you, so keep reading.

Keep reading and discover what normal sleep is, the challenges of sleeping in hot weather, evidence-based recommendations for summer sleep, and some unique tips you can apply to get better sleep in the summer and rest well during the scorching days and night.

GLOBAL WARMING

Without wanting to delve deep into global warming, I want to highlight some representative figures which are important to know, due to the implications not only on sleep, but the conservation of our planet, which is of great importance to us all.

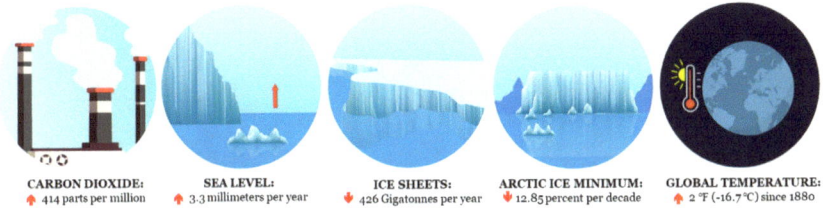

During the summer, temperatures are high, and they get higher every year as global warming and ambient temperatures increase. According to NASA Global Climate Change *(https://climate.nasa.gov/)* and National Centers for Environmental Information (NCEI), there's been a 2 °F (-16.7 °C) increase in temperatures since the industrial era (1880)[1]. Also, this increase has led to a rise in accumulated heat that affects not only the global land but also the oceans, with global surface temperatures having projected to expand by 0.5°C (0.9°F) in 2020.

That increase in heat has been of great disadvantage to summer sleep.

Moving on, before we discuss how to sleep like a baby during the summer and be well-rested when you wake up, let's start by getting an understanding of sleep, as this will form the basis of further discussions on sleeping in summer.

Let's begin.

Chapter 1: Normal Sleep: A Comprehensive Background

Chapter 1: Normal Sleep: A Comprehensive Background

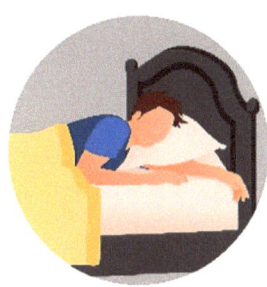

What structures in our brain are responsible for the occurrence of sleep? How do these structures work and how well are they working? What processes keep us asleep? What has to work so that we can sleep? What processes, what magic underlies our brain so that we can sleep?

If we wanted to answer in very brief words how our sleep-wake cycle works we could refer to the recent hypothesis of "fast-acting" neurotransmitters: Glutamate as a great booster of wakefulness and GABA (γ-aminobutyric acid) as the responsible and promoter of sleep (fig.1) [2].

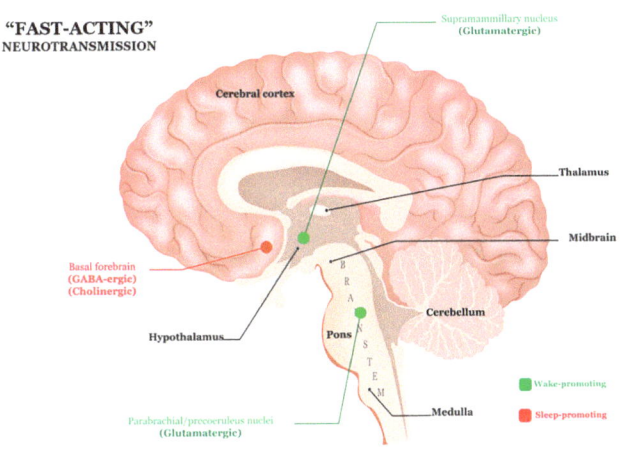

Fig. 1. Fast-Acting Neurotransmission

But the science behind sleep-wakefulness is more complex, as we will see.

Let's put it this way, it is impossible to tell if you're getting good sleep if you don't know what normal sleep feels like.

1.1 WAKEFULNESS

To start sleep, you have to be awake first. Our brain structures contain different cell groups (neurons) in charge of keeping us awake. It is not necessary to learn them by heart, but it is necessary to know that these regions exist, each of them in turn release a quantity of substances (neurotransmitters) that kept us balanced, maintain and regulate our consciousness to carry out our activities.

In general terms, the ascending reticular system (fig. 2) distributed by the brainstem releases noradrenaline, serotonin, dopamine, and histamine. There are also other brain structures such as the basal forebrain area and nuclei at the level of the pons in charge of releasing acetylcholine (fig. 3). All these substances, or neurotransmitters, play an active role in keeping us awake. However, some of them also participate to a lesser extent during sleep. Especially acetylcholine, which is also found in the REM sleep phase. Orexin/hypocretine substances produced in the posterior and lateral hypothalamus also acts as wakefulness and sleep regulators (fig. 4) [3].

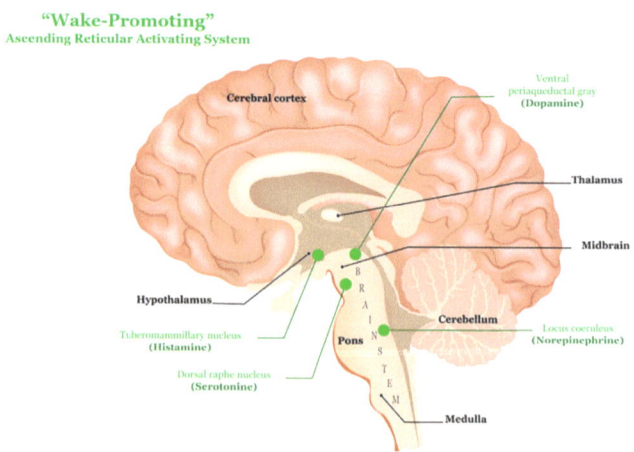

Fig. 2. Wake-Promoting. Ascending Reticular Activating System. Modulatory Monoaminergic Neurotransmission

Chapter 1: Normal Sleep: A Comprehensive Background

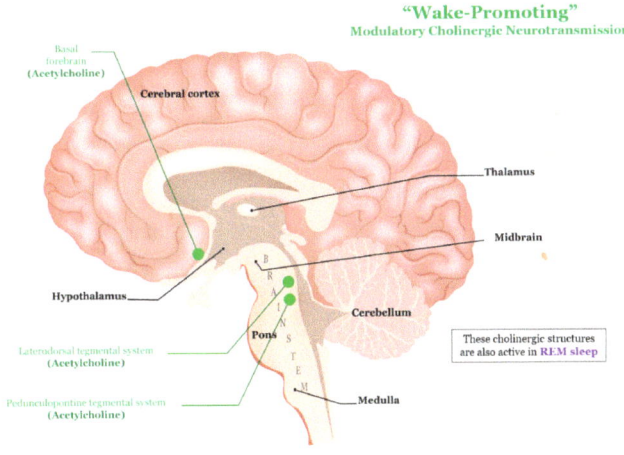

Fig. 3. Wake-Promoting. Modulatory Cholinergic Neurotransmission

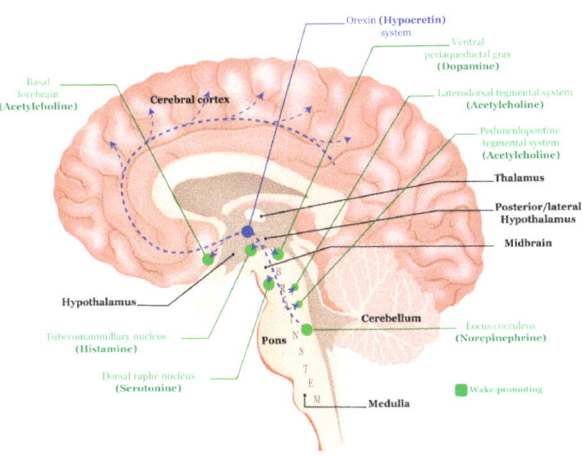

Fig. 4. Wake-Sleep Stabilizing. Orexin (Hypocretin) System

Chapter 1: Normal Sleep: A Comprehensive Background

All the brain activity originated by these neurotransmitters from these brain regions, are translated into waves also known as alpha activity that sleep specialists can see in the electroencephalogram (EEG) while you are awake.

In summer, some people worry that they have sleep issues when they don't fall asleep within 5 minutes of entering into this stage. However, you should be able to fall asleep within 20-30 minutes after you get into this stage. As we will see, there are many circumstances that prevent sleeping in the summer. But if you fall asleep almost immediately, maybe you are more than likely not sleep-deprived.

> **● ● ● Note**
>
> *Glutamate, serotonin, norepinephrine, histamine, dopamine, acetylcholine and orexin are modulatory neurotransmitters that promote wakefulness.*

1.2 SLEEP

Sleep is a physiological and behavioral process consisting of a decrease in the level of consciousness, with little response to external stimuli that occurs periodically, transiently and reversibly. We spend about 33% of our entire lives sleeping or trying to [4]. This becomes important if for instance we lived for 75 years, 25 years of our life would be spent sleeping. 25 years!!!

Everybody needs sleep, yet its principal organic reason stays remains a puzzle. Sleep influences pretty much every sort of tissue and framework in the body, from the brain, heart and lungs to digestion, and immunological capacity. However, an incessant sleep restriction, or poor-quality sleep, as is common in the summer or hot environments, leads to problems such as immune, inflammatory and cardiovascular [5].

A lot of people complain they're not getting enough sleep because they have certain expectations where sleep is concerned. They want to fall asleep immediately their head hits the pillow and not

Chapter 1: Normal Sleep: A Comprehensive Background

be interrupted until the next morning. Anything short of this is considered abnormal to them.

But that's not how sleep works.

Only through neurophysiological studies (EEG) is it possible to clearly recognize and differentiate the distinct phases that make up sleep (non-REM sleep and REM sleep) from wakefulness [6].

You also cycle between different sleep stages during your sleep (fig.5). Understanding this will help you get the most out of your sleep.

Let's spend some time looking at the various stages.

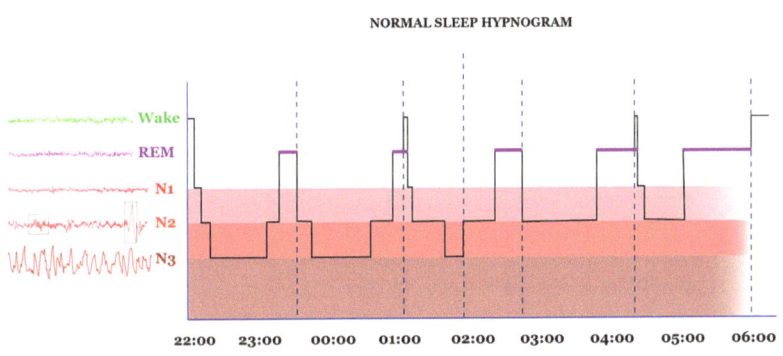

Fig 5. Normal Sleep Hypnogram. Through various sleep stages, a sleep cycle is usually around 90 minutes. In the first part, there is a progressive decrease in N3 (slow-wave) sleep. In the second part, there is an increase in the duration of rapid eye movement (REM)

Non-REM (NREM) Sleep

This part of sleep, under normal conditions, is usually the first part. It is around 75-80% of the amount of total sleep and comprises of stages N1, N2 and N3 [7].

Let's discuss the different stages of non-REM

Stage N1

Stage N1, is the changeover from wakefulness to sleep. Non-REM Stage 1 sleep usually lasts for 5 to 10 minutes and makes up for 3 to 8% of sleep time. In this stage, you're not yet fully asleep, but you're not fully awake either; rather, you're relatively awake and alert enough, that if someone were to wake you up, you'll easily claim that you weren't sleeping. Your brain will start to relax at this time. This is because your brain starts to produce slow brain waves known as theta waves. EEG in Polysomnography will indicate up to 50% reduction in the level of activity when you move from wakefulness to stage N1 sleep.

During this time, some people experience sudden jerks (sleep startles, hypnic jerks, predormital or hypnic myoclonus) and though the feeling is unpleasant, it represents a normal event during the transition from waking to sleep [8].

Stage N2

This is the second stage of non-REM sleep before you enter further deep sleep. When you enter this stage of sleep, eye movements are totally ceased, your body temperature drops and your heart rate and breathing slow down.

Something else that happens during this sleep stage, is that your brain starts having sleep spindles (bursts of rapid brain wave or electrical activity that are rhythmic). The type of sleep here is still light, and you tend to spend greater proportion of the total sleep time (about 50-60%) in this stage of sleep than in the other sleep stages [9].

Stage N3

I consider this to be the most important part of non-REM sleep and so I will go into more detail about it. This non-REM stage is the deepest stage of sleep that leads to you feeling refreshed when you wake up in the morning. Brain waves become regular and even slower, also known as delta waves. During the first half of the night, this stage of sleep will occur for longer periods if you had spent the whole of the previous day wake. Essentially this stage is characterized by your muscles relaxing, your breathing rate dropping and, your blood pressure dropping.

Stage N3 of sleep was previously categorized into stage 3 and stage 4, but recently, the stages were combined to form one stage. You spend about 13 to 23 % of your total sleep in a deep sleep.

When you're in non-REM stage N3, you become less responsive to the environment. Things such as noise and activity often fail to generate some type of response from you. If someone tries to wake you up, they'll find it harder to do so when you're in this stage of sleep.

People who are susceptible to sleepwalking, often do so when they enter this stage of deep sleep. When you are younger, you will have a deeper sleep. However, as you get older, it will become more difficult for you to go into a deep sleep. This is not because you need that kind of sleep less; rather, because your brain doesn't seem to be able to enter that kind of deep sleep. At an older age, sleep percentages change and sleep becomes more superficial with an increase in N1 and N2 [10].

Chapter 1: Normal Sleep: A Comprehensive Background

In a brain structural level, there is a reciprocal inhibition system between wakefulness and sleep. To initiate non-REM sleep, neuronal groups located in the anterior hypothalamus (ventrolateral preoptic area -VLPO-), inhibit the activity of the neuronal groups that are responsible for keeping us awake. The most recognized inhibitory neurotransmitter are GABA (γ-aminobutyric acid) and Galanine. These neurotransmitters are also produced in the thalamus, exactly in its reticular nucleus. Some of the waves recorded in the non-REM sleep phases originated from this region.

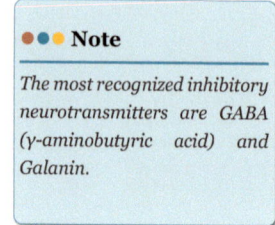

Note

The most recognized inhibitory neurotransmitters are GABA (γ-aminobutyric acid) and Galanin.

Another substance involved in non-REM sleep is adenosine. This substance has been related to sleep induction, especially when we have been awake for a long period of time. Adenosine reflects the energy expenditure of our brain during the day and is responsible for inhibiting areas of the brain that promote wakefulness. When we drink coffee to stay awake, we are avoiding increased sleep pressure on ourselves due to the accumulation of adenosine [11].

REM sleep

REM (Rapid Eye Movement) sleep is often thought to be the deepest stage of sleep, but it really is an active sleep, similar to being awake. You spend around 20 to 25 % percent of your total sleep time in REM sleep, and at this time your body is relaxed, your muscles immobilized, your brain becomes more active, your dreams are more vivid and your eyes experience rapid movement.

REM sleep is also known as paradoxical sleep. This is because, although your body systems and your brain become more active, your muscles are relaxed and immobilized. This prevents you from acting out your dream and causing harm to your body. It starts about 90 minutes after the onset of sleep, with the first period of the REM sleep taking about 10 minutes, and each recurring REM stage being longer than the previous one. The final one lasts about an hour. EEG waves patterns in REM sleep, seem pretty similar to wakefulness and sleep stage N1.

If you don't have any sleep disorder, you will experience increased and erratic patterns of respiration and heart rate. Moreover, your legs and fingers might twitch, and you will be more likely to have more dreams because of increased cerebral activity, all of which are accompanied by some sort of paralysis of the major voluntary muscles.

The most important neural groups for the onset of REM sleep are found in the brainstem. Above this region, nuclei located in the pons and in areas close to another region of the brainstem that

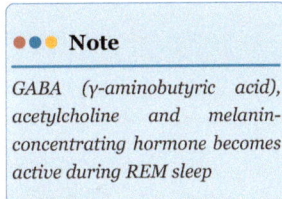

●●● **Note**

GABA (γ-aminobutyric acid), acetylcholine and melanin-concentrating hormone becomes active during REM sleep

is the midbrain are sufficiently active (called REM-on active cells) using acetylcholine as the fundamental neurotransmitter, which promotes a desynchronization of the activity of the cerebral cortex through the thalamus. Also, in the posterior/lateral hypothalamus, there are other REM-on active cells that produce both Melanin-concentrating hormone (MCH) and GABA, but unlike the exciting effects of orexins, both MCH and GABA are inhibitors. Another group of cells known as REM-off, which are minimally active in this phase of sleep, are also involved in the regulation of REM sleep. These REM-off cells use neurotransmitters that also participate in wakefulness (noradrenaline, serotonin, dopamine and histamine) and are located in the brainstem and prefrontal basal area [11].

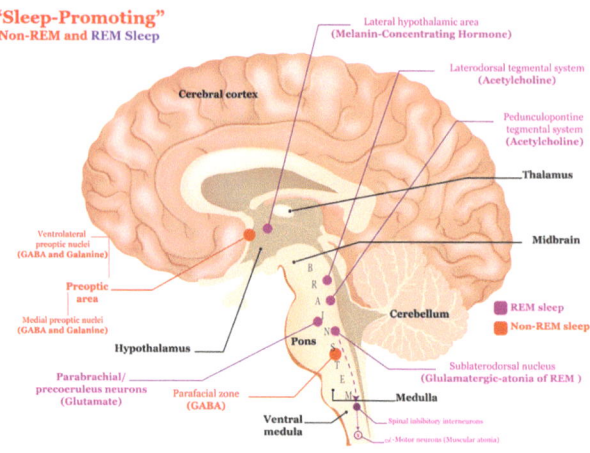

Fig 6. Sleep-Promoting Neurotransmission System

I understand that this part of the book is complex, and I hope you're following me. We have already gone through the most difficult part and if you are still with me I encourage you to continue to the most important part of this chapter which is the one that is most interesting in order to understand all the advice I will give you regarding sleeping in summer.

1.3 SLEEP MECHANISMS (THE TWO PROCESS-MODEL)

In summary, when it comes to the various stages of sleep, it is important to note that sleep is one side of the coin. We explain the other side of the coin by the hypothesis or model of the two processes. Your sleep drive is often referred to as Process S (Homeostatic) and your biological clock (circadian rhythm) is referred to as Process C (Circadian) [12].

Let's take a look at these two-processes model, and what they have to do with you enjoying optimal sleep.

Chapter 1: Normal Sleep: A Comprehensive Background

Process S (Homeostatic system)

The first thing you need to know is that Process S is the sleep drive [13]. It is a type of homeostasis.

What does this mean?

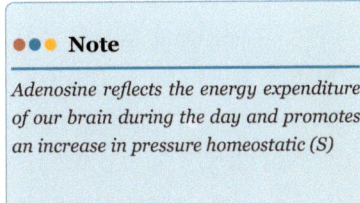

Note

Adenosine reflects the energy expenditure of our brain during the day and promotes an increase in pressure homeostatic (S)

Well, when loosely translated, the word homeostasis means 'same state'. In other words, homeostasis refers to the ability of living systems to maintain steady internal, chemical, and physical conditions. For example, you can have different types of homeostasis, such as regulation of blood sugar, regulation of temperature, surveillance of the immune system and sleep-wake homeostasis

The sleep-wake homeostasis basically refers to the way your body tends to incline towards sleep, once you've been awake for a certain period of time. The more hours you're awake, the more you'll feel the need to sleep.

In other words, think of starting the day with an empty backpack. As you go about your daily activities, you fill that backpack with different things (physical activities, household duties, professional occupations, problems etc.) As the day draws to an end, this backpack that was initially empty will now become full and heavy. This is the pressure of sleep. When you get home, what will you need to do? You will have to empty and release the accumulation in the backpack, and how do you do that? Well, you do so by sleeping. Sleeping helps you release that accumulated sleep pressure. The more things you accumulate throughout the day, the heavier the weight and burden to carry and the greater the need to free yourself from it. This is basically what the S or Homeostasis process is all about.

You can think of Process S, as some sort of timer; once you go without sleep, Process S reminds your body that you need to go to sleep.

When you take a short nap (around 20-30 minutes), you do not interfere with the way Process S regulates your sleep drive. This means that by evening, you should be able to go to bed, as usual. However, if you sleep for more than 30 minutes, then you'll enter into deep sleep stage N3, and this will prevent you from going to bed and sleeping instantly because you've already used up some of your needed sleep drive.

As such, you must be careful to only nap for a few minutes, if you don't want to stay awake when your bedtime arrives.

You may ask yourself now, why is it necessary for me to learn about anatomy, neurotransmitters, homeostatic process, and all these points...

Well, I hadn't told you, but sleep links homeostasis to the neuroplasticity processes of your brain. Neuro what????... Neuroplasticity. This is a process that takes place in your brain and involves the way your neurons strengthen the process they interact with (synapses). It covers the way neurons change and adapt to everything it exposes us to during the period.

What you learn, your experiences, your feelings, your brain picks these up, interprets and reacts to them, changing their structure and connections to keep work.

Neuroplasticity implies an effort, work, a waste of energy, a homeostatic weight that develops in wakefulness, increasing the load of those synapses in the brain circuits. Sleep decreases that synaptic load so that it is sustainable, and promotes while you rest, an efficient use of the space of the grey matter destined to work, especially for the benefit of learning and your memory. We could say that sleep is the price to be paid to keep neuroplasticity working properly, having as an aim through homeostatic regulation, to control the synaptic weight that affects the neurons (fig. 7).

According to this hypothesis, we can schematize it:

(1) When you are awake, there is an increase in the synaptic weight of our brain circuits and connections, because of the information to which we are exposed. This process has an energy expenditure, requires space and saturates the work process.

(2) An increase in the activity of slow waves in the brain through the EEG shows this synaptic weight is linked to homeostatic regulation.

(3) When synaptic weight decreases by homeostatic regulation, the slow-wave activity also decrease.

(4) The decrease of synaptic load linked to sleep effects, promotes an efficient performance of neuroplasticity processes, which translates into energy savings, use of space for these processes, benefits in learning and memory, a better capacity of synapses to maintain and strength in their connections.

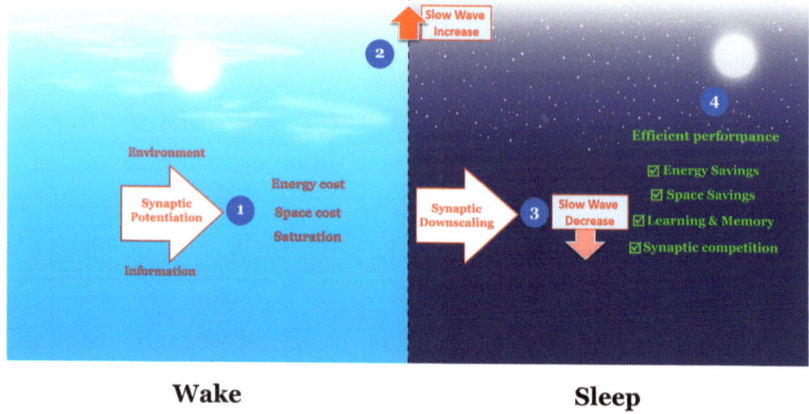

Fig 7. Functional implication of homeostatic sleep regulation

What about process C?

Process C (Circadian system)

We also know Process C as the circadian process or 'around the day' or 24 hours process. The term 'circadian rhythms' are usually used to refer to the inner biological clock.

Process C is driven by an endogenous pacemaker located in the suprachiasmatic nuclei of the hypothalamus. The plasma melatonin hormone and core body temperature are the most reliable markers of process C.

The function of melatonin is to help us prepare for the onset of sleep, melatonin is synthesized by the pineal gland, then released in the night and the levels stay high for several hours in order to stabilize sleep. When it is released, it increases its production in the evening with darkness, around 20:00 pm, then exhibits its highest peak in the middle of the night between 02:00 am and 04:00 am, then finally declines until levels fall in the early morning around 08:00 am [14].

Process C is a rhythmic activity that depends on the time of day or night and the biological clock, that is, what your body is used to.

The circadian rhythm is extremely useful because it is the one that dictates body functions. It dictates actions such as hormone release. It also regulates body temperature, brainwave activity, and communicates to you when you are feeling energetic, sleepy, or hungry.

But here's the thing. The process C is regulated by external signals (synchronizers, pacemaker, time givers or "Zeitgebers") [15]. Light is the most essential synchronizer, but there are other non-photic stimuli. For example, a regular caloric intake or social activities also participate in this process and its proper interaction and synchronization with the internal environment, leading to this process having an excellent performance. However, as we will see, in the summer we over-expose ourselves or abuse some of them.

Your biological clock is not cast in stone. Instead, it is flexible, and it resets each day. In another instance, let's say, when you fly to another area, you experience jet lag because your biological rhythm is out of sync with the new environment. It still ticks in tune with the time zone you left behind. However, after a while, your biological clock resets, and you are able to adjust to the new environment.

Your biological clock uses certain things each day. These include:

Light

One thing that resets your internal clock is light [16]. Your body knows to wake up due to the presence of light. Light, in this case, influences the production of melatonin; when the sun is shining, your body represses melatonin. This is the hormone responsible for making you sleepy, and it is produced when it is dark. Thus, the presence of light and low melatonin levels signify it is time to wake up.

However, it's not just sunlight that affects your sleep pattern. Blue light also affects your sleep.

This is the type of light that is found in items such as:

- Smartphones
- Gaming systems
- Television
- Tablets
- Computer monitors
- LED bulbs
- Fluorescent light bulbs

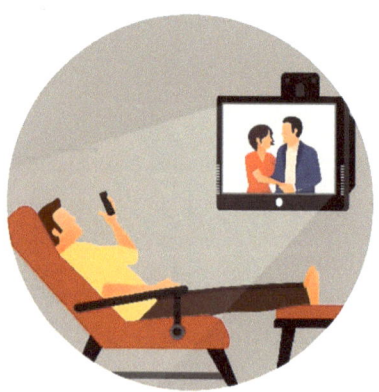

Exposure to such items disrupt your sleep, because your eyes can't block such light well. As a result, when you keep using various items that emit blue light, the light passes through to your retina in a bid to enable your brain translate the light into the different images. In other words, your brain will be fully awake as it takes in the images you're constantly providing it with.

But there's another reason why blue light disrupts your sleep.

As we've said, your body needs darkness to produce melatonin. Thus, when you keep using blue light at night, you are just preventing yourself from going to sleep since your body

●●● **Note**

Melatonin helps us sleep. It is released in the dark 2 hours before bedtime, and reaches a maximum value 2 to 3 hours before waking up. Exposure to screens with blue light (electronic device screens) suppresses this hormone

is prohibited from producing melatonin, which works to make you sleepy. Keep in mind that all forms of light – whether sunlight or blue light, suppress the production of melatonin. Thus, to reset your circadian, you need to limit your exposure to blue light and increase your exposure to sunlight during the daytime.

Now let's look at something else that affects your biological clock.

Meals

If you notice, another of the things Process C or your internal clock tells you is when you're hungry. If you've trained your body to expect food late into the night, for example, in the case of late-night snacking, it will definitely alert you when it is time to eat.

Unfortunately, when you consume a meal close to bedtime, it ends up interfering with the winding down process. Unhealthy eating habits impact your sleep [17]. This is because, food needs to be digested and absorbed into your body. Meaning once you eat something late into the night, your body is going to be busy trying to use up what you've given it. This keeps you awake for longer.

But apart from the time you eat interfering with your sleep, what you eat can also keep you awake.

If your diet is full of highly processed foods, too much sugar, and high in carb, it will mess up your sleep pattern. Such foods make you feel drowsy and fatigued. As such, they interfere with your daily routine, and you end up dozing off when you shouldn't. This in turn, affects your sleep at night.

Thus, if you change up the food you eat and the time you eat it, you'll be able to reset your biological clock.

Social interactions

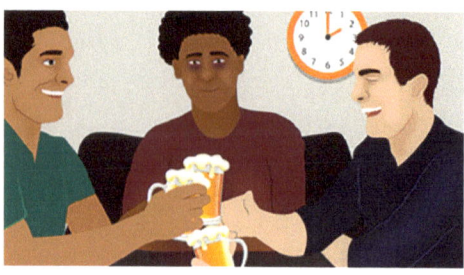

Social interactions are important to your life, but they are another factor that impacts your internal clock [18]. While you're busy chatting with friends and living it up at night, you're eating into the time for your sleep. Thus, you end up going to bed late, and this makes you fail to wake up early. In case you do set an alarm clock to enable you to wake up early, you'll still need to deal with sleep debt as you cannot cheat nature, and your body will still feel as if it has not rested.

But it gets worse.

Since you're sleepy, you may decide to give in and catch up on the sleep you lost at night. This worsens the situation as it prevents you from going to sleep later on that night, and the problem starts all over again the next morning. Thus, if you want to reset Process C, you need to keep an eye on your social interactions.

These three things can help you reset your biological clock to where you want it to be and this will help you sleep better at night.

> ●●● **Note**
>
> *Your sleep drive is Process S (Homeostatic) and your circadian rhythm is referred to as Process C (Circadian). They control and adapt your sleep to the needs of the organism.*

So, how are Process C and Process S related?

Process S and Process C work together to create your sleep-wake cycle (fig. 8). For example, when you feel tired at night, your sleep drive (Process S) happens to be the strongest, and Process C (circadian) boosts it by releasing melatonin. Melatonin is produced when it's dark, and is responsible for making you sleepy. Thus, at night, both Process S

Chapter 1: Normal Sleep: A Comprehensive Background

and Process C work together to enable you to get some sleep.

So, what happens if Process C and Process S are not well-aligned?

When these two processes are well-aligned, you feel well-rested because you're able to get enough sleep. On the other hand, if they are not well-aligned, you may end up suffering from social jet lag. This is a state that signifies different sleep-wake times from those of society. In other words, you'll find yourself waking up too late and going to bed too late. In turn, you may have issues performing your daily tasks, especially if they are supposed to be done during the morning hours. Moreover, you may be sleepy throughout the day.

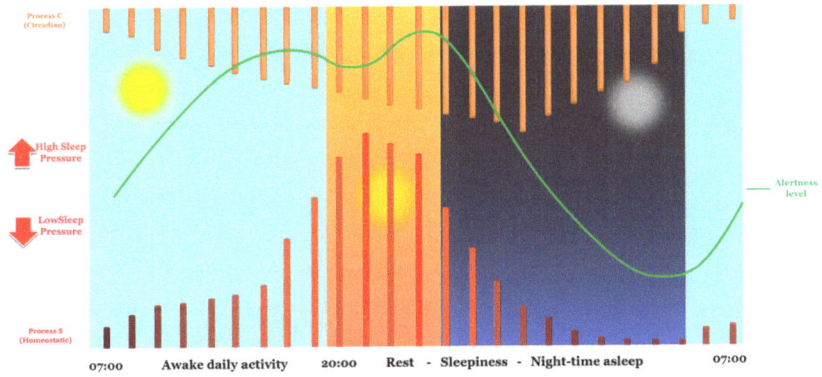

Fig 8. Two-Process model of sleep

Thus, your biological clock needs to work well if you wish to enjoy optimal sleep.

Unfortunately, various issues may make it hard for you to sleep in the summer or during the hot weather, and these might throw off your internal clock. Let's look at some of the challenges you may face.

> ●●● **Note**
>
> *Healthy sleep depends on a complex interaction of substances and brain structures that regulate and ensure the sleep-wake cycle is continuous and stable.*

Chapter 2: Challenges To Sleep In Summer Or Hot Weather

Chapter 2: Challenges To Sleep In Summer Or Hot Weather

2.1 SEASONAL EFFECTS ON SLEEP

Despite the progress in different fields of scientific research in sleep medicine, it has not yet been possible to establish a direct relationship on the influence of the different seasons on sleep quality. Most of the studies that have been done, focused on a pattern of depression, present in the fall and winter seasons that is relieved during the spring or summer months and is known as Seasonal Affective Disorder. This is good news for the summer.

However, there are some studies that have shown a relationship between the change of seasons and some sleep problems. It has been 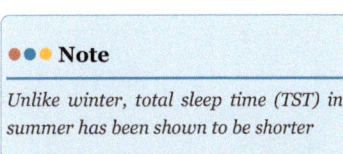 shown that in some regions, the duration of sleep is influenced by the seasonal change. During the winter, the sleep time was longer and during the summer the sleep time was shorter. These changes are more significant in middle-aged and older people, with little impact on younger people. It is a fact that, during the months of spring and summer, there is a greater difficulty in falling asleep, maintaining sleep and a higher possibility of early morning awakening [19, 20].

> **Note**
> Unlike winter, total sleep time (TST) in summer has been shown to be shorter

Furthermore, it is important to note that, during the seasons, the amount of light varies between different geographical positions. As we have seen, light is an important sleep regulator. In this sense, a study was carried out which showed that the duration and quality of sleep are not strongly affected by the season. Instead, it is the insufficient exposure to daylight from areas inhabiting polar regions that has a major influence on sleep onset latency, efficiency and duration [21]. In summer, daytime is longer in some areas, with more exposure to light, and this seems to be another piece of good news for our dream. But as we will see later, not all that glitters is gold.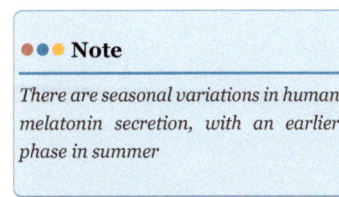

> **Note**
> There are seasonal variations in human melatonin secretion, with an earlier phase in summer

2.2 SUMMER SLEEP DISRUPTORS

Apparently, the effects summer has on our sleep don't seem to be so damaging. In an ideal world, nothing would be able to interfere with your internal balance and your internal clock. As such, when both homeostasis and your circadian rhythm are well-balanced, you would have no issues falling asleep.

But as you know, the world is not perfect. The weather is not perfect, and your body is not immune to interference. Thus, several things in the summer or related to a hot weather, can interfere with your sleep. Some of which include:

Long Days

Summer is that time of year when the days get longer and the nights get shorter. During the summer, it is not unusual to have 14 hours of daylight on a good day. Some places get up to 19 hours of daylight, come the summer solstice. That is a lot of daylight!

But the thing with daylight is that it is associated with certain activities.

When it is bright outside, you want to be outside. You want to do things you can't do when it's dark. Also, many people love taking advantage of the summer to get in as many activities as they can. They want to let loose and enjoy themselves, and who can blame them?

But what this results in, is later sleeping time.

This is especially so since staying up later usually translates into eating food later. And we've seen already, how this interferes with your sleep pattern.

Chapter 2: Challenges To Sleep In Summer Or Hot Weather

Hot Nights (the temperature effect)

In relation to light, it seems that the temperature is another important regulator of the duration and time of sleep [22].

The temperature, as we saw before, depends on the endogenous control of the circadian rhythm, and this aspect is fundamental to being able to sleep. It has been known for a long time that when we go to sleep, a drop in body temperature is essential to start sleeping [23].

Our body temperature fluctuates throughout the day. Body temperature begins to drop from approximately 36.5 °C (97.7 °F) at midnight. It approaches 36 °C (96.8 °F) around 04:00 hours. From this time, body temperature begins to increase again, exceeding 37 degrees Celsius (98.6 °F) after noon (12:00) and reaching a maximum of 37.5 °C (99.5 °F) between 17:00 and 18:00 hours, dropping again to between 36.5 and 37 °C (97.7 to 98.6 °F) at midnight. The drop that occurs from 18:00 hours in body temperature is what makes us sleepy [24].

As far as most people are concerned, it's not yet summer until the weather is hot. Unfortunately, this also translates into the night, and rarely do hot nights and sleep get along. While you're busy tossing and turning because it's too hot, you're also not getting any sleep.

When the hottest day of summer arrives, you might as well give up on getting any sleep if you don't have ways to counteract the temperature. But why is it so hot during the summer solstice? Well, it is hot because of the buildup of heat. Weeks before the solstice, the amount of solar energy hitting the ground is often more than that leaving the earth as seasonal lag hits.

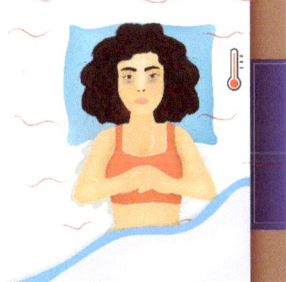

Chapter 2: Challenges To Sleep In Summer Or Hot Weather

Vacation Jet Lag

In relation to temperature, jet lag alters the relationship between slow wave sleep activity and thermoregulation, causing difficulties not only in initiating and maintaining sleep, but also causing a disruption in the architecture of sleep and daytime performance when we are awake [7, 25]. Jet lag travelers experience rapid change over the circadian system leads to an asynchrony in endogenous oscillatory components (out of phase) with the environment [26]. It can also be compared to the social jet lag that many people who sleep late normally experience. Think about it. What happens when you go on vacation? First, you may end up traveling to a different time zone, and this causes jet lag as your body insists on remaining in the old time zone. Second, you want to hit the ground running and such, you neglect to rest up and lastly, you want to use up every opportunity to get the most of every penny you spend. This means late nights and early mornings. Is it any wonder that you may experience difficulty sleeping during the summer?

Too Much Alcohol

The thing with alcohol is that it does make you sleep more quickly at first, but you'll get to enjoy deep sleep only for a while [27]. Eventually, it will wear off and once it does, instead of enjoying a restorative sleep, you'll find yourself waking up suddenly.

Unfortunately, during the summer, many people do not spend a lot of time being cautious of their alcohol intake. This is especially so if they're on vacation. They use that opportunity to overindulge in all the vices they don't get to indulge in during other seasons.

Thus, their sleep pattern gets messed up, and they find it difficult to stay asleep through the night.

Chapter 2: Challenges To Sleep In Summer Or Hot Weather

Alcohol also happens to worsen the symptoms of sleep apnea. If you use it regularly, not only will you find it difficult to sleep later on at night, but you may also end up exhibiting issues such as sleep talking and sleepwalking.

Spicy Foods

Spices make you enjoy your food and appreciate different flavors and cultures. This is something many people look forward to when they visit various places. But when the food is spicy, it tends to impact your sleep because it can cause digestive issues such as heartburn.

Even if you're spared from heartburn, there is something else you need to know about spicy food.

Spices such as red pepper are responsible for increasing your core body temperature [28]. However, when you sleep, your core body temperature tends to drop. Therefore, if it was too high to begin with, your body will have a difficult time adjusting to the temperature transition, and this will interfere with your sleep.

It's also good to note that eating a variety of foods can cause you to experience other digestive issues such as bloating and constipation. Thus, if you're going to experiment with different cuisines during the summer, you have to be careful about how you go about it.

Afternoon Naps

It has been clearly recognized, that napping decreases the accumulation of the homeostatic pressure of sleep when we go to sleep (remember the backpack full of things). It's not uncommon for people to snooze during the daytime come summertime. This is especially so, if they'd been enjoying a variety of activities during the morning. You may want to 'catch up' on sleep during

Chapter 2: Challenges To Sleep In Summer Or Hot Weather

the afternoons, but it's good to remember that naps are only useful when they are taken for a few short minutes [29].

If you spend a lot of time napping, you'll disrupt your sleep pattern, and this will have a domino effect as you'll always be struggling to catch up on your sleep as you sleep late and wake up late.

Mosquitoes and Other Bugs

Mosquitoes and bugs love the summer. The way they buzz about taking a bite out of people, you'd think they wait for summer just to have a huge biting party. Worse still, they don't remain quiet while biting you. They buzz away and interfere with your sleep. You're either busy swatting at them away or waving your hands, trying to chase them away. This also interferes with your sleep.

When they eventually bite and you start scratching away, you may end up feeling more uncomfortable as your skin becomes inflamed. Worse still, if the scratching leads to open wounds, you'll have a hard time controlling it and finding that restful sleep.

If you don't have a screen on your window, you need to invest in one and check on it from time to time to ensure it does not have gaps that can allow bugs in.

Allergies

Seasonal allergies tend to cause people to sneeze a lot. During the summer, allergies can bring forth a variety of unpleasant symptoms, such as runny nose, sneezing, watery eyes, cough, postnasal drip, allergic shiner, adenoidal or allergic face, fatigue, nasal crease and mouth breathing due to nasal congestion.

Summer allergies are often mistaken for other ailments such as food intolerances or colds.

Chapter 2: Challenges To Sleep In Summer Or Hot Weather

Summer allergies are often triggered by pollen, specifically grass pollen. Grass pollen is distributed via the wind. Thus, on warm, windy days, it gets to affect millions of people, and when you're suffering from various symptoms due to allergies, you find it difficult to fall asleep [30]. This is especially so if your symptoms become worse due to summer air pollution.

Lack of Deep Sleep

Deep sleep is the type of sleep that makes you feel rested. Unfortunately for many people, summertime is that time of the year they fail to stay asleep long enough to enjoy deep sleep.

Think about it.

As we've said, there are several reasons why people fail to fall asleep during the hot season. Now, take those reasons and imagine them causing you to wake up at different times at night.

If you've just fallen asleep and just as you're about to fall into deep sleep, you're abruptly woken up because your allergies are acting up or a mosquito is on the rampage or the alcohol is no longer in your system, or your sheets are too sweaty, you'll have trouble going back to sleep again. Then when you eventually do go back to sleep, something else may end up waking you up.

Expectedly, by the time you wake up, you feel as if you didn't rest at night. This results in you wanting to sleep during the day, and in turn, disturbs your sleep at night. The cycle could go on like this.

Lack of Exercise

Many people don't like exercising, let alone exercising in the hot weather. But even those who love exercising give themselves a break from exercising during vacation. After all, they've been working

Chapter 2: Challenges To Sleep In Summer Or Hot Weather

hard throughout the other months and feel as though they deserve a break. Unfortunately, when you laze about throughout the day, you don't do yourself any favor. Exercise is said to improve sleep and reduce insomnia [31].

Thus, you shouldn't neglect it just because you are on vacation.

Poor Sleep Hygiene

As you know, your bed should be used for sex and sleep alone, and many people follow that rule of thumb. But as soon as summer arrives, that rule gets thrown out of the window. Instead of going to bed just to sleep, you may end up eating in bed, reading, watching television, or just hanging out with your friends or family as you tell stories late into the night. In the end, all these bad habits ensure that your sleep is of less quality and duration, also causing a dehydration that in summertime, can affect or worsen our renal function [32].

Importantly, once your brain gets used to such things, you'll find it harder to go to sleep. This is because your brain no longer recognizes your sleep routine. Instead of it starting to wind down as soon as you enter your bed, it will still be wide awake because it no longer gets the signal to wind down.

Poor Air Quality and Humidity in Our Room

It seems that this is an issue that we hardly ever think about when we go to sleep. We generally underestimate the air quality (oxygen and carbon dioxide levels) of our external environment, the thermal conditions and indoor air quality (IAQ). I don't think we closely examine the humidity conditions either. At least air pollution is being taken into account in the last few years. These are all situations that in one way or another, also affect our quality of sleep.

Chapter 2: Challenges To Sleep In Summer Or Hot Weather

Let's see how.

Air pollution as an external factor, acts as a significant sleep disruptor. It has mainly been shown to be associated with obstructive sleep apnea. Optimal oxygen levels at the brain level stimulate deep and restful sleep. When oxygen levels are low, sleep becomes unstable and unsynchronized, remaining in a state similar to that of being awake. In some cases, inducing that our brain during sleep remains longer in REM sleep. High levels of pollution cause irritation of the airways. Entry of small particles through the lungs into the bloodstream, and even the added psychosocial aspects increase the risk of obstructive sleep apnea by 60% [33].

Some international guidelines state that for a fresh air supply to exist in an indoor area, CO_2 concentrations must be below 1800 mg/m3 (1000 ppm). However, there are frequent clinical manifestations or complaints (fatigue, headaches and increased heat perception of unpleasant odours at concentrations as low as 1100 mg/m3 (600 ppm) [34]. For various reasons (closed rooms to maintain privacy, absence of windows, energy savings in air conditioning, etc.), especially in hot and humid regions, rooms are not always well ventilated, and it is often possible to find CO_2 levels above 2500 ppm. In these conditions it is possible to find alterations in the quality of sleep by increasing the frequency of awakenings and decreasing the efficiency of sleep. Fortunately, it is possible to decrease the concentration of CO_2 to between 55% and 64% by opening the bedroom door while sleeping. This simple measure significantly improves our quality of sleep, makes our bedroom cooler and makes us feel less sleepy during the day and more able to concentrate so that we can enjoy the summer [35, 36].

Finally, Humidity. Humidity is defined as the amount of water vapor suspended in the air. There are three types of humidity (absolute, relative and specific). We are interested in knowing the relative humidity (relationship between air humidity and saturated humidity). It has been considered that for a proper and healthy environment, humidity should be between 40% and 60%, which is achieved with temperatures close to 22 °C (71 °F) or about 20-24 °C (68-75.2 °F). However, it is necessary to adapt these values to the period of the year or the external environment in which we find ourselves. Additionally, it is important to note that exceedingly high humidity levels are just as disruptive as low humidity levels. When the humidity is higher in your room, it is more difficult for the humidity to evaporate from your body, therefore, you feel hot, uncomfortable, and sweaty. High humidity encourages the growth of mould, which can trigger allergies and breathing problems in response to the inflammatory reaction triggered by allergy, leading sleep problems and even respiratory disorders. On the other hand, low humidity levels cause dryness in the airways, skin, eyes and hair of people and continuing this harmful dryness, makes it easier for microorganisms to enter our bodies increasing the risk of infection [37].

All in all, there are a variety of reasons that people have trouble sleeping during the summer. Fortunately, there are also a variety of things you can do to improve your sleep, even if the weather is hot.

> ••• **Note**
>
> The most important disruptors of summer are bad sleeping habits, sudden alteration of the circadian rhythm, lack of deep sleep, high humidity, poor air quality and of course the effect of high temperature.

Let's look at science-backed strategies that will help you sleep better, beat insomnia and rest on hot days and nights this summer.

Chapter 3: Evidence-Based Recommendations For Summer Sleep

Chapter 3: Evidence-Based Recommendations For Summer Sleep

Before we delve into what you can do to improve your sleep during the summer, it is important to understand why you need sleep in the first place, because once you understand that, you'll see why you need to put in the effort to get better sleep.

Sleep is important because it:

- ☑ Increases concentration and productivity
- ☑ Lowers the risk of unnecessary weight gain
- ☑ Makes the immune system stronger
- ☑ Improves athletic performance
- ☑ Improves heart health
- ☑ Prevents depression
- ☑ Lowers inflammation
- ☑ Leads to steadier blood sugar levels and
- ☑ Boosts your mood

Thus, it is in your best interest to improve the quality of your sleep. But as we've seen, the challenges that come with summer can interfere with your sleep. In any case, with challenges often come solutions, and that's what we want to concentrate on.

Some things you can do to sleep better in the summer include:

3.1 DON'T NEGLECT YOUR SLEEP SCHEDULE

A lot of people assume that they sleep less during the summer. Thus, they tend to brush off any symptom that there could be a problem with their sleep, but what do evidences show?

Chapter 3: Evidence-Based Recommendations For Summer Sleep

Well, according to a study, people tend to sleep less during the summer than they do during other months of the year, with winter being the time they sleep the most [19]. But get this, the difference between summer sleep and winter sleep is less than 12 minutes, and when it came to all the seasons, only older people showed a significant difference when it came to sleep during various seasons. They slept more than other age groups.

So, what is the take out for you?

It means that you should not neglect your sleep simply because it is summertime. The idea that you need less sleep or you should go to bed at unreasonable hours just because it is summer, is not supported by science.

However, when summer arrives, you find people going to bed later than they would if they were not on vacation. For example, parents often allow their kids to stay up one or two hours later, and kids begin to expect it whenever summer arrives. But as we've seen, the difference between summer and winter sleep is, on average less than 12 minutes. Thus, if you wanted to stay within those limits, you would go to bed only 12 minutes later than you would during other times.

The point is that you need to maintain your sleep schedule during all seasons. You need to determine:

Your Wake-Up Time

The first step to creating a great sleep schedule is to determine the time you need to wake up. Think of all the things you do each

> ●●● **Don't neglect your sleep schedule**
>
> *Even on vacations and weekends, keep your sleeping and waking hours fixed. If you take naps, reduce their duration to less than 30 minutes. After 3:00 in the afternoon, don't take naps, and at night don't go to bed until you are sleepy. Finally, if you cannot fall asleep within 20 minutes, get up and try a quiet activity. Don't return to bed until you feel sleepy.*

morning and the activities and chores you have to accomplish, then give yourself enough time to do them without hurrying too much. Next, determine your sleep time.

Your Sleep Time

To determine your sleep time, you need to ask yourself how many hours you need for sleep. If you need seven or eight hours, you have to work backward to determine when you'll be going to bed. Once you do that, you have to make sure you're in bed at that time each day, even during the weekends or holidays.

The idea is to train your body to respond to certain bedtime cues once your sleep time arrives. That way, your internal clock adjusts to your sleep-wake cycle, and you'll have made a crucial first step when it comes to getting better sleep during summer.

3.2 CONTROL LIGHT SOURCE EXPOSURE

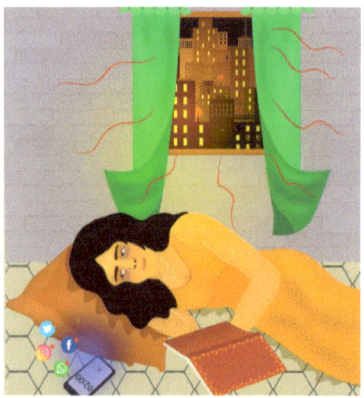

Light influences everything from metabolism to body temperature and sleep. Sunlight triggers the production of serotonin. This is a hormone that works to boost your mood and help you feel calm and focused. Thus, it is important you get some sunlight in the morning as this will help you regulate your sleep.

However, if you know you'll be outside for more than 15 minutes, you should remember to put on some sunscreen. The summer sun can be harsh on your skin. You don't want to get skin issues all because you were trying to get some sun.

Chapter 3: Evidence-Based Recommendations For Summer Sleep

But as we've said, during summer, you are exposed to prolonged daylight, and this suppresses the production of melatonin, the sleep hormone that works to make you sleepy. This suppression is great when it is morning. However, the body needs to start producing melatonin as the day goes by to prepare you for sleep at night. Let's be clear the duration of your sleep is affected by your circadian rhythm, which is affected by your melatonin levels. In turn, your melatonin level is affected by your exposure to sunlight [38].

Thus, you must get enough sunlight each day.

Now, let's look at blue light. As already mentioned, blue light negatively impacts your sleep.

Thus, you need to:

- Block out blue light with a pair of glasses – You can use a pair of glasses to block blue light. Amber, brown-tinted or red-tinted lenses could work perfectly. However, they tend to distort colors and thus need some time to get used to.

- Turn off your screens – You need to cut back on using various devices two or three hours before your sleep time. This will help prepare your brain for sleep.

- Install filtering apps – You can install apps to filter blue light on your computer screen, tablet and smartphone. This way, your eyes will not be exposed to a lot of blue light. Some of

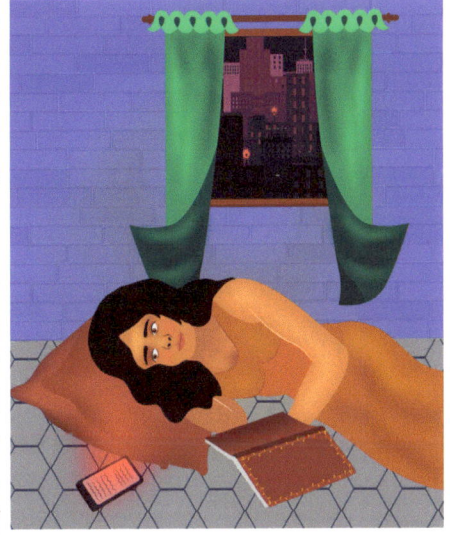

Chapter 3: Evidence-Based Recommendations For Summer Sleep

the popular apps include: F.Lux, Redshift, SunSetScreen, Iris, Twilight and more

- Dim your lights – Something else you can do is put your devices in dark mode or night mode, as this will darken your display background and lessen your exposure to blue light.

- Change your light bulbs – Some bulbs give off more blue light than others. For example, incandescent bulbs use up a lot of energy and emit more blue light than LEDs and fluorescent bulbs. Fluorescent bulbs emit less blue light than LEDs. Thus, if you were to choose, you should go for fluorescent bulbs.

- Use red night lights – If you wish to have a night light, you should use a red light bulb. This is because the color red is less harmful to your circadian rhythm.

Apart from being smart about blocking out blue light, you need to remember that the light outside is something you can control from getting inside your home. As such, once your bedtime is approaching and it is still bright outside, you can use your curtains or drapes to block out the light.

> ●●● **Control light source exposure**
>
> *Block out blue light with a pair of glasses (amber, brown-tinted or red-tinted lenses). Stay away from electronic device screens and use light filters widely known in the market (F.Lux, Redshift, SunSetScreen, Iris, Twilight, and more)*

Remember also to stop using electronic devices two hours to your bedtime. This will give you the best chance at experiencing improved sleep. Now let's look at another way you can improve your sleep.

Chapter 3: Evidence-Based Recommendations For Summer Sleep

3.3 REGULATE YOUR INTERNAL TEMPERATURE

What does temperature have to do with sleep?

Well, it has a lot to do with it. This is because you cannot enjoy a good night's sleep if the temperature is too hot or too cold. For you to enjoy your sleep, the temperature needs to be about 16-18 °C (60-64 °F).

But just how important is the temperature?

Well, for the longest time, people thought that sleep patterns were only affected by things such as light. They assumed that people who did not have access to night light would be able to stay asleep till morning. However, one study focusing on a hunter-gather community in Tanzania threw that assumption out of the door.

The study of 33 men and women of the Hadza tribe found out that the members of the community tended to wake up at various points in the night [22]. Their being awake was linked to temperature rather than the time of night. This goes to show the importance of regulating temperature, especially during the summer period.

Other studies support the claim that the thermal environment is a significant factor in human sleep [39].

According to the study, exposure to heat increases wakefulness. It also works to decrease REM sleep. People who sleep nude or semi-nude are more affected by exposure to cold than exposure to heat. Thus, it is important to choose your sleep clothes and bedding wisely.

Another thing to note when it comes to temperature, is that your core body temperature tends to decrease when you are experiencing nocturnal sleep. It also tends to increase during the wake phase, and these instances are repeated throughout the 24-hour circadian rhythm.

You are more likely to go to sleep when your core body temperature decreases.

The good news is that there are things you can do to bring your core body temperature down when you want to go to sleep. Some of the things you can do to regulate your temperature include:

3.4 CHOOSE NATURAL FIBERS

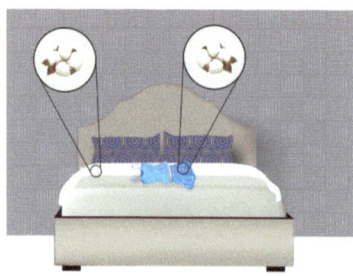

Natural fibers such as fiber flax have unique thermal qualities that are ideal for sleeping conditions, no matter the climate. Though, fiber flax is better to use in warm temperatures, especially for is heat conductivity. Fiber flax has 5 times more heat conductivity than wool and 19 times more heat conductivity than silk. With fiber flax, the human body temperature is kept 3-4 degrees Celsius lower than with silk or cotton. In addition, in terms of economy, elements made from linen have a durability of more than 20% (linen becomes stronger when wet, by a factor of about 20%), compared to other materials, which wear out with each wash.

Cotton sheets also work better in the summer because they happen to be breathable. Meaning if you sweat at night, you won't have to wake up due to sweaty sheets.

Choose fiber flax or cotton instead of silk, satin, or polyester and get rid of heavier coverings as they'll only bring in more heat [40, 41].

> ••• **Choose natural fibers (fiber flax and cotton)**
>
> *Choose clothing or bedding made of natural fibers (flax fiber or cotton). Do not use synthetic materials.*

3.5 TRICK YOUR SHEETS

Something that can help you bring down the temperature is cool sheets. You can place your sheets in an airtight plastic bag and then place the bag in a freezer. This will allow your sheets to stay cool. Remove them just before you go to sleep.

You can also spritz your sheets with water. Keep the spritz bottle near your bed so that you can sprinkle more water on your sheet during the night if the need arises.

3.6 USE A COLD WATER BOTTLE

Cold water bottles come in handy whenever you want to soothe your muscles. They can also be useful when you want to cool down, you just need to freeze some water in the bottle and then place it in your pillow. This will help to cool down your core body temperature.

A buckwheat pack can also be used to cool down. Freeze it for some time and when the time comes for you to sleep, put it in your pillow for the best results.

3.7 KEEP YOUR FEET AND HANDS OUT

When it's hot at night, you can cool down by ensuring that your feet and hands are hanging out of the covers. You can go a step further and tuck in the sides so that you don't get tangled in your sheets. Remember, the idea is to lose heat from your hands and feet, and this means they should be at a lower temperature than the rest of your body. Don't wear any socks on your feet as this will be counterproductive.

3.8 CHECK YOUR SLEEPWEAR

Some people argue that it is better to sleep nude to keep the heat off, while some argue that you need to wear pajamas so that when you sweat, they can soak up the moisture. The choice is yours, but if you choose to wear pajamas, you should choose a fabric that is designed to wick humidity away. For example, a bamboo-viscose blend does this well. Alternatively, you can wear loosely woven fiber flax or cotton to bed.

3.9 WET YOUR PULSES

An excellent way to keep cool, is to use cold compresses or herbal cooling towels on your pulses. You should place the compress inside your elbows, behind your knees, at the base of your neck, around your groin, and on your wrists. Applying the compress at pulse points on your ankles and wrists can bring you great relief.

3.10 SOAK YOUR FEET

You can soak your feet if you need quick relief from the heat.

Here is how to go about it:

Pour some cold water to a bucket and place your feet inside for a few minutes before you go to bed. You can keep the bucket of water close to your bed in case you want to use it later on at night.

3.11 USE A FLANNEL

If you wish to cool down at night, the secret is to keep your head cool and your body warm. You can do this by placing a wet flannel on your forehead. First, you need to place the flannel in the refrigerator and let it stay there for an hour, before using it on your forehead right before you go to sleep.

Chapter 3: Evidence-Based Recommendations For Summer Sleep

The thing with flannels is that you need to dip them in cold water once they start getting warm. As such, you can store some cold water in a thermos and use it to wet the flannel whenever you need to do so.

3.12 USE A RICE SOCK, THERMIC SEED BAGS OR GEL PACKS

This involves placing raw rice inside an old sock. Once it is filled up, use an elastic band to tie the opening of the sock to hold the rice in place. After that, place the rice sock in the freezer for several hours. This way, you can use it to cool your neck and face when you go to bed at night. If you want, you can have several rice socks so that you can apply them to your hands as well. There are also Thermic Seed Bags or Gel Packs available in the Market or you can make them yourself following the instructions on the web.

3.13 MIST A COOLING SPRAY

The hot air circulating through the night can easily mess up your sleep. As such, you need to find ways to cool it down. You can do this by adding some water into a spray bottle. Place the bottle in your fridge and then use it to spray water into the air from time to time. You can also use a mixture of half water and half alcohol. This way, the water will evaporate faster due to the alcohol, and this will help you cool down.

If you wake up in the middle of the night due to the heat, you can use the cooling spray on your face and neck; this will also help you cool down.

3.14 USE A FAN

A standing or ceiling fan can be your greatest ally when you're working to improve the quality of air within your home. It can keep the air circulating so that you're not forced to breathe in hot, stale air. Place the fan on a table near your bed or put it at the end of your bed. This will stop you from getting too hot as you sleep. Also, it doesn't hurt that the gentle humming noise of the fan can help soothe you to sleep.

You can try to determine the direction the wind is blowing from to know where to position the fan. Many people place the fan right at their bedroom window when they want cool air to blow into the room, although you have to ensure the cool air is actually blowing inwards before you leave the fan there.

3.15 ICE THE AIR

Sometimes using a fan is not enough to cool down the air. At such times, you can go a step further and use ice to cool down the temperature some more. Start by filling a tray with ice and then add a bit of water into the tray. Next, place the fan behind the ice tray. This way, the fan will be able to blow cool air in your direction as the ice melts.

The good thing about ice is that it takes a while to melt. Thus, you'll experience cooler temperatures for a while as the fan blows the cooled down air into the room.

Note: it would be a good idea to keep a supply of ice cubes handy in case you want to change the water in the tray.

3.16 REFRAIN FROM COLD SHOWERS

When you are feeling hot, it is really tempting to take a cold shower to cool down. But while the water is cold, it does nothing to help you in the long run. This is because taking a cold shower works to raise your body temperature, and this makes it harder to sleep. Rather than taking a cold shower, you can run your wrists and feet under

Chapter 3: Evidence-Based Recommendations For Summer Sleep

some cold water for a few minutes, as this will help you cool down.

If you want to take a shower, you should take warm baths - not too hot not too cold. Of course, you'll feel warm as you shower, but after a while, your body will cool down, and this will bring the core body temperature down, helping you have an easier time falling asleep.

All in all, remember that cooling your core body temperature will help you sleep better.

Now let's look at another way you can improve your sleep.

3.17 IMPROVE THE THERMAL CONDITIONS AND INDOOR AIR QUALITY (IAQ).

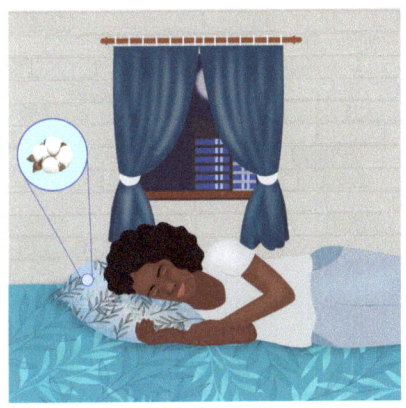

When we talk about summer sleep, it would be prudent to mention the role summer pollution plays in the disruption of sleep. When summertime comes, the incidents of sleep-disordered breathing increase [42]. This is mainly due to the pollutants that are rampant during summer. Thus, when you want to improve your sleep, it would help to reduce your exposure to air pollution.

Worth mentioning is the difficulty in separating air pollution and temperature when it comes to respiratory problems. For example, studies that have been done in Europe, show that there are associations between increased respiratory mortality and high temperature. Humidity is another issue.

Chapter 3: Evidence-Based Recommendations For Summer Sleep

When the temperature is high, you tend to sweat a lot. Unfortunately, humidity makes it really hard for the sweat to evaporate and thus hinders the cooling effect that stems from sweating. Fortunately, there are some things you can do to improve the air you breathe in. You should:

3.18 OPEN THE DOORS AND WINDOWS

When it's hot, it helps to keep the windows and doors open. This way, a cool breeze can get through and help cool down the temperature. Bugs are however a huge problem when the weather is hot. Consequently, you have to find a way to lock them out or shut your windows at dusk. Another alternative is to invest in a mosquito net for screening the windows, gazebos, patios, porches, etc. This way, you can keep your windows open even at night, to keep the air cool and fresh.

3.19 VENTILATE THE ATTIC

In your quest to cool down your home, you need to remember that hot air rises. This means, it has a chance of escaping if only it had a way of doing so. You can provide that way by opening the hatch on your attic. If you do this, the hot air will escape, and the temperature in your room will cool down. Remember as well to open your bedroom doors, to allow the trapped hot air escape.

3.20 MOVE ROOMS

When you sleep upstairs, you'll feel the heat. This is because of the hot air, which tends to rise. Hence, if you want to cool down, you can should downstairs where the temperature is lower. If you have kids, you can arrange an 'indoor camp' for them and move everyone downstairs so that all of you can escape from the heat.

Chapter 3: Evidence-Based Recommendations For Summer Sleep

3.21 KEEP THE STOVE OFF

Summertime is the time to do as little cooking as possible, inside your kitchen. If you wish to cook, it would be better to use the grill outside. If you must cook inside, you should turn on the fan and keep your windows open. This way, the hot air can quickly escape as it forms.

If you have to use the stovetop, you should make sure that your windows are open.

3.22 USE A DEHUMIDIFIER

At times, the muggy air is more of a hindrance to sleep than the hot temperature. The humidity level should be about 30 to 50 percent. Therefore, if you're struggling with humidity, you may want to get a dehumidifier to keep things in check throughout the summer.

3.23 GET OUTSIDE

Fresh air and sunlight are vital for your sleep, but you have to be careful when you go outside during the day due to the effects of UV rays. Stay safe, stay prepared, and ensure you apply sunscreen. The sunlight will be great for regulating melatonin, and so, when evening approaches, you'll be able to get the sleep you want.

There may be a reason you have to go outside at night.

As much as you may wish to stay in your home, it may not be practical to continue doing so if the place is too hot and humid. This is especially so if you have a shady yard you can use. You can get out of your house and sleep outside to escape the hot air inside.

In some countries, you could find that there is a cooling center in your neighborhood [43]. This way, if things get too uncomfortable,

Chapter 3: Evidence-Based Recommendations For Summer Sleep

you can quickly head to the cooling center and save yourself from having a heatstroke. When you take the time to change the things you can change, you'll find yourself not only sleeping at night, but also being able to improve the quality of your sleep.

It would be a good idea to keep a packed bag ready so that you can quickly move to a different area in case the weather changes abruptly. Remember to pack some water in the bag because you may have to wait for a bit before you get your hands on a bottle of water.

> ●●●**Regulate your internal/ external temperature**
>
> *Remember that your core body temperature must drop to start sleep. Do not do intense physical activity for at least 3-4 hours before going to bed. The perfect room temperature is between 16-18 oC and 60-64 oF. Humidity levels should be between 40% and 60%.*

Now let's look at some other things that can help improve your summer sleep.

Chapter 4: Other Related Tips

To get better sleep during hot nights, some other things you should do are:

4.1 CHECK YOUR DIET

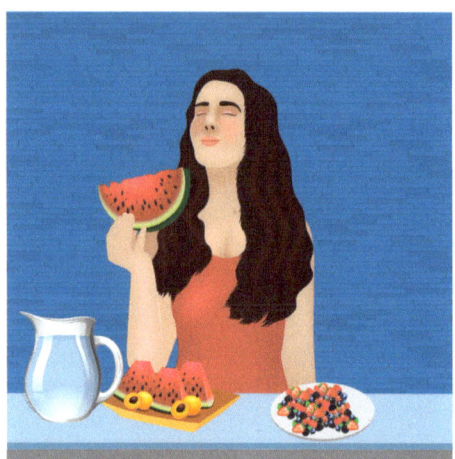

One way to make your life easier during the hot and humid summer is to consume cooling foods. Now is not the time to cook hot meals on your stove, rather, a time to invest in something chilled. Therefore, you should make it a point to plan your meals with foods that don't require much preparation.

Hydrating foods such as cucumbers, go a long way in cooling you down and ensuring you don't become dehydrated [44]. You can eat raw cucumbers, add some slices in your water, prepare a chilled cucumber soup, or add some cucumber slices to your salads. This will ensure you stay hydrated throughout the day.

Something else you need to include in your diet is dark greens. Foods such as lettuce have high water content, and they can be used in sandwiches and salads. Remember, you're trying to avoid cooking whenever you can. Thus, equipping yourself with vegetables that you can use in your salads and sandwiches should be your first priority.

You can use vegetables and fruits to prepare different types of smoothies, and add some cubes into your drink to keep it chilled. The good thing about this is that you avoid cooking, but you still get to eat healthy. Hence, the sleep issues that come with overindulging

Chapter 4: Other Related Tips

in unhealthy foods will not be an issue for you.

Fruits such as berries, peaches, grapefruit, and watermelon are in season during the summer. Why not take advantage of such foods and use them well throughout the summer? You'll be able to enjoy the different tastes, cool down, and avoid adding heat to your home by eating them.

If you crave for something to eat, you should try eating grilled cheese, sandwiches, chilled soba noodles, steak and salad, eggs on toast, and cold vegetable salads. There are many combinations of food you can enjoy throughout the summer. A good meal plan will give you variety and make eating such foods a joy.

Apart from checking your diet, you also need to check the time you eat.

Many people throw the rule book out of the window when it comes to eating during the summer. They may start the day late and finish it late, and this means eating late into the night. As you well know, if you eat late into the night, you'll have trouble sleeping. This is especially so if you indulge in heavier foods.

So, what should you do?

You should determine what time of the day is cooler and schedule your heavier meals around that time. For example, during the summer, it is not unusual for the morning hours to be cooler. Hence, you can decide to start your day by eating a heavy breakfast and then stick to salads and soups for the rest of the day. The idea is to be done with eating heavier meals a few hours to your bedtime.

> ●●● **Check your diet**
>
> *Maintain a balanced diet low in carbohydrates and sugars. Stay hydrated. Fruits such as berries, peaches, grapefruit, and watermelon are in season during the summer.*

Not only will this keep you cool, but it will also prevent you from gaining that vacation weight that so many people complain about at the end of their vacation.

4.2 STAY HYDRATED

When the weather is hot, you tend to sweat a lot, and this means you risk getting dehydrated if you don't drink a lot of fluids.

The most important fluid you can drink is water. Water is useful in regulating your body's temperature and preventing you from getting dehydrated. Therefore, you have to keep it close to you all the time. You should:

- Start your morning with several glasses of water – If you want to drink more water daily, you'd better start off your day right by consuming one or two glasses of water. Make it a habit to do this, and you'll soon be doing it without much thought. But remember, you shouldn't be too quick to gulp down the water immediately you wake up. This may cause you to bring it back up. Instead, drink it slowly and give it time to settle in your stomach.

- Keep a glass nearby at mealtimes – A lot of people drink soda, beer or wine with their meals. That is all well and good, but those beverages cannot give you the benefits that drinking a glass of water can. If you stick to drinking water, you'll be able to stay cool, not just for a few minutes but for hours. Remember, water protects you from becoming dehydrated. It cannot be compared to other drinks.

- Have several water points – You shouldn't have to head to the kitchen to have access to drinking water. Rather, you should have several water points around your home, so that you are always reminded to drink water whenever you see it. Also, if you want to spend some time outside, put some bottles of water in a cooler box and make sure you drink them from time to time.

Chapter 4: Other Related Tips

- Add flavor to your water – Fruits such as watermelon, lemon, and cucumber add different flavors to your water. This makes it easier to drink several glasses of water without getting tired of drinking water or feeling as if you're drinking too much water. This is especially so if your water has a funny taste. Sometimes people avoid drinking water because of the way it tastes or because they can't detect any taste from it.

All in all, when it comes to water, remember not to wait until you're thirsty to reach for a glass. This is because, by the time your body signals you that it is thirsty, you're already dehydrated. Drinking enough water throughout the day ensures that you don't get to that state.

4.3 LIMIT SOCIAL INTERACTIONS IN THE EVENING

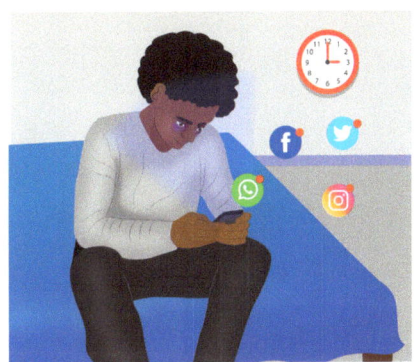

Summertime is a good time to socialize and meet new friends. However, you need to schedule your time well so that you don't spend a lot of your evenings interacting with other people, such that you disorganize your sleep schedule [18].

Instead of scheduling such interactions in the evenings, you can schedule them during the day or early in the evening. Try to finish social interactions at least two hours before your bedtime. And yes, this includes chatting with friends on various social media platforms.

If you have a family living with you, you can use that time before you go to bed to get to know them better.

> ●●● **Limit social interactions**
>
> *Try to finish social interactions at least two hours before your bedtime. And yes, this includes chatting with friends on various social media platforms.*

Tell each other stories instead of watching television shows, and then ensure that you go to bed as per your sleep time.

4.4 EXERCISE

Exercise impacts your sleep at night, and it can come in handy when you are dealing with sleep issues such as insomnia [45].

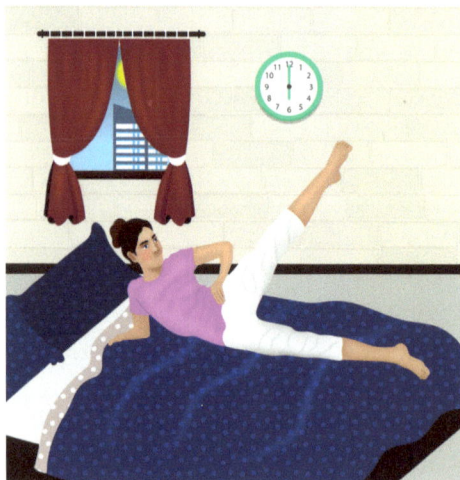

However, during summer, the very idea of exercising in the hot weather is enough to induce a headache, but this should not prevent you from exercising. Think of it as an adventure and schedule various activities that you can do to get a full-body workout. For example, instead of running indoors, you can switch to swimming. This way, you'll get to enjoy the water and still get the much-needed exercise.

As you plan to exercise, you should plan to do so several hours before your bedtime. This is because you tend to increase your core body temperature when you exercise. So, exercising close to your bedtime will not help you cool down. And as you exercise, you need to drink some water so as not to get dehydrated. You want to improve your sleep, not fall down in a faint.

Chapter 4: Other Related Tips

4.5 HANG CLOTHES OUTSIDE

When the weather is hot, it is time to switch off your washing machine and dryer and start doing laundry outside.

Think about it; during winter, you end up putting some clothes on indoor drying racks because you can use the dryer to dry them. Now, imagine doing so during the summer. That is just a recipe for increasing humidity in the air.

However, if you hang the clothes on an outside drying rack or hanging lines, they'll not only dry faster but you'll also not have to deal with humidity. Before you go hanging clothes outside, it would be wise to see if there are any restrictions. Various neighborhoods usually have different bylaws with regards to such things.

4.6 CLEAN YOUR GUTTERS

When it's hot, you don't need to add moisture to your home again, because this will just increase the humidity unnecessarily, and you'll have to deal with hot, muggy air. So, what can you do to prevent this from happening? Well, the first thing you can do is to examine your pipes to see if any of them are leaking. If you find any leakage, you need to make sure you repair them or wrap up the pipes using insulators. The idea is to stop the leaks from adding moisture to your home.

You also need to ensure that you clean your gutters. This is because gutters often contribute to water leakages.

4.7 SLEEP IN A HAMMOCK

When your bed becomes too hot to sleep in, you can look at alternatives. A hammock is one thing that can help you ditch your bed. You don't have to go outside, you can just tie it somewhere in your room. The good thing about sleeping in a hammock, is that you'll have better air circulation than you would have if you'd slept in a mattress. Additionally, you'll also get to benefit from the sleep spindle effect that comes with the gentle rocking motion of a hammock.

4.8 USE COOLING/MIGRAINE PATCHES

The thing about heat is that it brings forth various complications. One of the complications is frequent headaches. To cool your head down, you can make use of migraine patches. These cooling patches are specifically designed to cook your head quickly and consequently, allow your core body temperature to come down. You can place the patches on the back of your neck and your body. You can also place them on other areas that feel very hot. In these cases, always take into consideration the information given by your neurologist or your family doctor.

4.9 NEVER FORGET YOUR MEDICATION

Keep in mind that during the summer, there are some illnesses that can get worse. It is important to never forget to take your medicines at the right time. It is common to travel and forget your medication at home, so make sure your medication is the first thing you put in your travel bag. Keep your health insurance up to date in case something unexpected happens. If you use a CPAP device for your obstructive sleep apnea syndrome, take it with you and wear it at least 4 hours a day.

4.10 TRY A WOOL MATTRESS TOPPER

If you wish to cool your bed, you have to look into things such as the type of mattress you have, your bed coverings and your sheets. During summer, you'd want to use coverings that can wick moisture away quickly and keep you cool. Wool is one breathable material. It not only absorbs moisture, but releases it to allow you to stay cool. Therefore, you should think about getting a mattress covering made from wool instead of sticking with foam. Remember that other materials such as fiber flax and cotton are also recommended.

4.11 UNPLUG YOUR ELECTRONICS

It's good to remember that your electronics and lights give off heat [46]. Thus, it is not enough to just switch off your electronics; you also need to unplug them from the sockets to prevent them from generating heat. If you want to make your work easier, you can plug the electronics into a power strip. This way, you'll have fewer things to unplug as you cool down your home.

4.12 INVEST IN DESICCANTS

When you want to cool your home, invest in a dehumidifier or in desiccants. Desiccants are usually available in dollar stores or hardware stores. You can buy them in buckets and store them at various points in your home. This way, they'll be able to suck out the moisture wherever you place them.

However, you'd want to place them in an area where kids or pets cannot reach them.

4.13 LISTEN TO THE RAIN

There is something soothing about listening to the rain. This is because your brain recognizes the sound of the rain as non-threatening. As you know, the rain does not fall down on cue, and as such, you have to get creative. One thing you can do is to download the sound of rain and use this 'pink noise' to ease yourself to sleep. The sound of rain can improve the amount of time you spend in deep sleep, and this goes a long way in making you feel rested.

It's also important to note that a lot of people associate rain with cold weather. Hence, listening to the sound of rain may actually trick your brain into believing that you are enjoying a cool weather.

4.14 TRY PRANAYAMA

Did you know that you can cool your core body temperature by the way you breathe? This is possible using a cooling exercise known as Sitali Panayama. This yoga exercise involves sitting down in a yoga position, with your spine, neck, and head aligned and your legs folded [47]. Hold each hand on top of a knee with the thumb touching the pointing finger.

Next, form an O shape with your mouth as you open it, and then stick your tongue past your upper lip. Once done, pretend you're drinking something through a straw as you proceed to breathe in slowly via your mouth. Next, close your mouth and proceed to breathe out via your nostrils. Repeat the breathing exercise for about 2 to 3 minutes. This should cool you down.

Remember, you don't have to wait to get hot to practice Pranayama. You can do so at at any time of the day.

4.15 MAINTAIN PROPER SLEEP HYGIENE

Sleep hygiene is something that comes up now and then whenever the topic of a lack of sleep is discussed. The bottom line is that if you want to enjoy decent sleep, you must work on your sleep hygiene.

What does sleep hygiene encompass?

Sleep hygiene encompasses a lot of things we've already touched on. These include:

Chapter 4: Other Related Tips

- Determine how many hours you need to sleep - Everyone is different. If you're getting enough sleep, you shouldn't need an alarm clock to wake up.

- Sleep in a quiet place – Your room should be as quiet as possible. Figure out how to shut out the noise and refrain from playing loud music as you go to bed.

- Choose your sleep time and stick to it – A regular sleep time will train your body to anticipate sleep as the time draws near.

- Don't misuse your bed – Your bed should only be used for sex and sleep. This means all other activities should be done in a different place. Also, you should avoid having other furniture other than your bed in your bedroom, as much as possible.

- Keep your room dark – Use curtains or drapes to keep your bedroom dark. If there is a lot of heat outside, refrain from opening the curtains in the morning. This will keep the room cool.

- Limit screen time – As evening approaches, you will need to stop spending so much time on electronic devices. The light emitted from such devices can further disrupt the quality of your sleep.

- Don't nap for long – You should limit the amount of time you spend on napping to avoid messing up your night sleep.

- Watch your diet - You should watch what you eat and determine when you'll eat it.

- Limit caffeine and alcohol – Watch what you drink as it can mess up your sleep.

- Adhere to a bedtime routine - A good bedtime routine helps prepare your brain for help.

Chapter 4: Other Related Tips

- Remember do exercise to improve your sleep

- Calm down—Keep daytime problems away from bed and sleep.

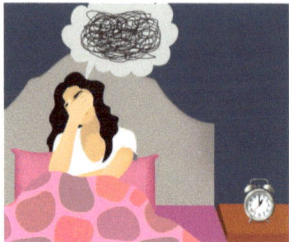

Everyone has problems. If you have a lot of problems and they go around in your head, a good option is to write them down in a notebook on your bedside table. This way, your brain will associate that you are paying attention to them and that when you are more rested the next day, you will be able to solve them.

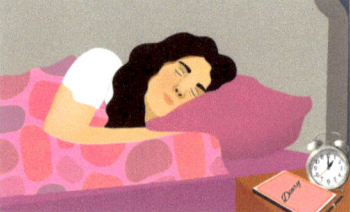

As you can see, there are several ways to improve your sleep during hot weather. Some of them you probably already knew, and others from the contents of this guide. The most important thing is to have a combination of things that work for you and use them throughout the summer to your benefit.

> ●●● **Don't take your problems to bed.**
>
> *Calm down. Keep daytime problems away from bedtime and sleep. Write down your problems or thoughts in a notebook on your bedside table. The next day, when you are well rested, you will think better about how to solve them.*

That said, if in spite of following all these recommendations and trying everything over and over again, you continue to have problems in maintaining an adequate quality of sleep (accompanied by other clinical manifestations such as intense headache on waking, excessive daytime sleepiness or fatigue and poor energy throughout the day), I would recommend that you go to a doctor specialized in sleep disorders near your city of residence or visit an online physician recognized with credentials. He/She would be able to evaluate and offer you the specific treatment that best suits your particular situation.

CONCLUSION

Summertime does not lessen the importance of sleep, but it just may make it harder for you to sleep well if you don't take precautions. This is why you need to know the various things you can do to sleep well and rest up during the summer or hot weather.

We've learned a lot about the sleep cycles and why they matter in your quest to dealing with summer sleeplessness, the different unique challenges that come with summer that increase the chances of having trouble sleeping as well as powerful evidence-based approaches towards dealing with summer sleeplessness. It is likely you've been able to identify several explanations that explain the challenges you've been dealing with.

Don't just gather the information; use it for your benefit to ensure summer is no longer the season when you have to struggle with sleep year in year out. Yes, there is a way out of your challenges and this book has detailed everything you need to do to find your way out.

If you follow the tips outlined, you'll no doubt enjoy good sleep, no matter the weather condition.

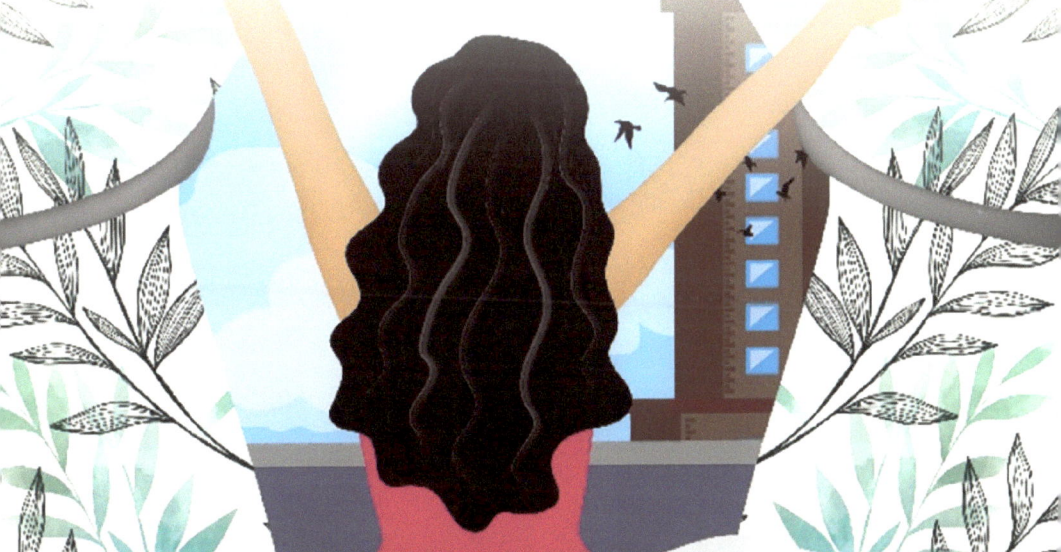

REFERENCES

1. *National Centers for Environmental Information (NCEI), State of the Climate: Global Climate Report for Annual 2019, published online January 2020, retrieved on January 16, 2020 from https://www.ncdc.noaa.gov/sotc/global/201913*

2. *Saper CB, Fuller PM. Wake-sleep circuitry: an overview. Curr Opin Neurobiol. 2017;44:186-192. doi:10.1016/j.conb.2017.03.021*

3. *España RA, Scammell TE. Sleep neurobiology for the clinician. Sleep. 2004;27(4):811-820.*

4. *Aminoff MJ, Boller F, Swaab DF. We spend about one-third of our life either sleeping or attempting to do so. Handb Clin Neurol. 2011;98:vii. doi:10.1016/B978-0-444-52006-7.00047-2*

5. *Faraut B, Boudjeltia KZ, Vanhamme L, Kerkhofs M. Immune, inflammatory and cardiovascular consequences of sleep restriction and recovery. Sleep Med Rev. 2012;16(2):137-149. doi:10.1016/j.smrv.2011.05.001*

6. *Berger, H. Über das Elektrenkephalogramm des Menschen. Archiv f. Psychiatrie 87, 527–570 (1929). https://doi.org/10.1007/BF01797193*

7. *Chokroverty, S. (2017). Overview of normal sleep. In Sleep disorders medicine (pp. 5-27). Springer, New York, NY.*

8. *Oswald I. Sudden bodily jerks on falling asleep. Brain. 1959;82(1):92-103. doi:10.1093/brain/82.1.92*

9. *Berry, R. B. (2011). Fundamentals of Sleep Medicine*

E-Book: Expert Consult-Online and Print. Elsevier Health Sciences.

10. Olini, N; Huber, R (2014). Ageing and sleep: sleep in all stages of human development. In: Bassetti, C; Huber, R. ESRS Sleep Medicine Textbook. Regensburg: European Sleep Research Society, 73-82.

11. España RA, Scammell TE. Sleep neurobiology from a clinical perspective. Sleep. 2011;34(7):845-858. Published 2011 Jul 1. doi:10.5665/SLEEP.1112

12. Borbély AA. A two process model of sleep regulation. Hum Neurobiol. 1982;1(3):195-204.

13. Colten HR, Altevogt BM, Institute of Medicine (US) Committee on Sleep Medicine and Research, eds. Sleep Disorders and Sleep Deprivation: An Unmet Public Health Problem. Washington (DC): National Academies Press (US); 2006.

14. Cajochen C, Kräuchi K, Wirz-Justice A. Role of melatonin in the regulation of human circadian rhythms and sleep. J Neuroendocrinol. 2003;15(4):432-437. doi:10.1046/j.1365-2826.2003.00989.x

15. Duffy JF, Wright KP Jr. Entrainment of the human circadian system by light. J Biol Rhythms. 2005;20(4):326-338. doi:10.1177/0748730405277983

16. Blume C, Garbazza C, Spitschan M. Effects of light on human circadian rhythms, sleep and mood. Somnologie (Berl). 2019;23(3):147-156. doi:10.1007/s11818-019-00215-x

17. Nakajima K. Unhealthy eating habits around sleep and sleep duration: To eat or fast?. World J Diabetes. 2018;9(11):190-194. doi:10.4239/wjd.v9.i11.190

18. Kent RG, Uchino BN, Cribbet MR, Bowen K, Smith TW.

Social Relationships and Sleep Quality. Ann Behav Med. 2015;49(6):912-917. doi:10.1007/s12160-015-9711-6

19. *Suzuki M, Taniguchi T, Furihata R, et al. Seasonal changes in sleep duration and sleep problems: A prospective study in Japanese community residents. PLoS One. 2019;14(4):e0215345. Published 2019 Apr 18.*

20. *Putilov AA. Retrospectively reported month-to-month variation in sleeping problems of people naturally exposed to high-amplitude annual variation in daylength and/or temperature. Sleep Sci. 2017;10(3):101-112. doi:10.5935/1984-0063.20170019*

21. *Friborg O, Bjorvatn B, Amponsah B, Pallesen S. Associations between seasonal variations in day length (photoperiod), sleep timing, sleep quality and mood: a comparison between Ghana (5°) and Norway (69°). J Sleep Res. 2012;21(2):176-184. doi:10.1111/j.1365-2869.2011.00982.x*

22. *Yetish G, Kaplan H, Gurven M, et al. Natural sleep and its seasonal variations in three pre-industrial societies. Curr Biol. 2015;25(21):2862-2868. doi:10.1016/j.cub.2015.09.046*

23. *Henane R, Buguet A, Roussel B, Bittel J. Variations in evaporation and body temperatures during sleep in man. J Appl Physiol Respir Environ Exerc Physiol. 1977;42(1):50-55. doi:10.1152/jappl.1977.42.1.50*

24. *Thomas KA, Burr R, Wang SY, Lentz MJ, Shaver J. Axillary and thoracic skin temperatures poorly comparable to core body temperature circadian rhythm: results from 2 adult populations. Biol Res Nurs. 2004;5(3):187-194. doi:10.1177/1099800403260620*

25. *Harding EC, Franks NP, Wisden W. The Temperature Dependence of Sleep. Front Neurosci. 2019;13:336. Published 2019 Apr 24. doi:10.3389/fnins.2019.00336*

26. *Vosko AM, Colwell CS, Avidan AY. Jet lag syndrome: circadian organization, pathophysiology, and management strategies. Nat Sci Sleep. 2010;2:187-198. Published 2010 Aug 19. doi:10.2147/NSS.S6683*

27. *Stein MD, Friedmann PD. Disturbed sleep and its relationship to alcohol use. Subst Abus. 2005;26(1):1-13. doi:10.1300/j465v26n01_01*

28. *Nisar M, Mohammad RM, Arshad A, Hashmi I, Yousuf SM, Baig S. Influence of Dietary Intake on Sleeping Patterns of Medical Students. Cureus. 2019;11(2):e4106. Published 2019 Feb 20. doi:10.7759/cureus.4106*

29. *Hilditch CJ, Centofanti SA, Dorrian J, Banks S. A 30-Minute, but Not a 10-Minute Nighttime Nap is Associated with Sleep Inertia. Sleep. 2016;39(3):675-685. Published 2016 Mar 1. doi:10.5665/sleep.5550*

30. *Centers for Disease Control and Prevention (CDC), 2017. https://www.cdc.gov/nchs/fastats/allergies.htm*

31. *Kline CE. The bidirectional relationship between exercise and sleep: Implications for exercise adherence and sleep improvement. Am J Lifestyle Med. 2014;8(6):375-379. doi:10.1177/1559827614544437*

32. *Rosinger AY, Chang AM, Buxton OM, Li J, Wu S, Gao X. Short sleep duration is associated with inadequate hydration: cross-cultural evidence from US and Chinese adults. Sleep. 2019;42(2):10.1093/sleep/zsy210. doi:10.1093/sleep/zsy210*

33. *Billings ME, Gold D, Szpiro A, et al. The Association of*

Ambient Air Pollution with Sleep Apnea: The Multi-Ethnic Study of Atherosclerosis. Ann Am Thorac Soc. 2019;16(3):363-370. doi:10.1513/AnnalsATS.201804-248OC

34. Government of Canada: Health Canada Exposure Guidelines for Residential Indoor Air Quality. April 19987. Revised July 1989. Available online: http://publications.gc.ca/collections/Collection/H46-2-90-156E.pdf

35. Mainka, A.; Zajusz-Zubek, E. Keeping Doors Closed as One Reason for Fatigue in Teenagers—A Case Study. Appl. Sci. 2019, 9, 3533. doi: 10.3390/app9173533

36. Strøm-Tejsen P, Zukowska D, Wargocki P, Wyon DP. The effects of bedroom air quality on sleep and next-day performance. Indoor Air. 2016;26(5):679-686. doi:10.1111/ina.12254

37. Özdamar Seitablaiev, Melek & Umaroğulları, Filiz. Thermal comfort and indoor air quality. international journal of scientific research and innovative technology. Vol 5. No. 3, pp 90-109, 3, 2018.

38. Choi JH, Lee B, Lee JY, et al. Relationship between Sleep Duration, Sun Exposure, and Serum 25-Hydroxyvitamin D Status: A Cross-sectional Study. Sci Rep. 2020;10(1):4168. Published 2020 Mar 6. doi:10.1038/s41598-020-61061-8

39. Okamoto-Mizuno K, Mizuno K. Effects of thermal environment on sleep and circadian rhythm. J Physiol Anthropol. 2012;31(1):14. Published 2012 May 31. doi:10.1186/1880-6805-31-14

40. Abitha M, et al. "Thermal Conductivity of Fabrics." Applied Mechanics and Materials, vol. 813–814, Trans

Tech Publications, Ltd., Nov. 2015, pp. 768–772.

41. Frydrych I, Dziworska G, & Bilska J (2002). Comparative analysis of the thermal insulation properties of fabrics made of natural and man-made cellulose fibres. Fibres and Textiles in Eastern Europe,2002, 10(4), 40-44.

42. Zanobetti A, Redline S, Schwartz J, et al. Associations of PM10 with sleep and sleep-disordered breathing in adults from seven U.S. urban areas. Am J Respir Crit Care Med. 2010;182(6):819-825. doi:10.1164/rccm.200912-1797OC

43. Pacific Gas and Electric Company (PG&E) Cooling Center locations. https://www.pge.com/en_US/safety/emergency-preparedness/natural-disaster/heat/cooling-centers.page (last access august, 2019)

44. Popkin BM, D'Anci KE, Rosenberg IH. Water, hydration, and health. Nutr Rev. 2010;68(8):439-458. doi:10.1111/j.1753-4887.2010.00304.x

45. Brupbacher G, Straus D, Porschke H, et al. The acute effects of aerobic exercise on sleep in patients with depression: study protocol for a randomized controlled trial. Trials. 2019;20(1):352. Published 2019 Jun 13. doi:10.1186/s13063-019-3415-3

46. Fuller C, Lehman E, Hicks S, Novick MB. Bedtime Use of Technology and Associated Sleep Problems in Children. Glob Pediatr Health. 2017;4:2333794X17736972. Published 2017 Oct 27. doi:10.1177/2333794X17736972

47. Bankar MA, Chaudhari SK, Chaudhari KD. Impact of long term Yoga practice on sleep quality and quality of life in the elderly. J Ayurveda Integr Med. 2013;4(1):28-32. doi:10.4103/0975-9476.109548

ABOUT THE AUTHOR

Dr. Fredy A. Escobar Ipuz is an author, clinical neurophysiologist, expert in sleep medicine an active researcher with a passion for helping people improve their sleep patterns and enjoy the refreshing benefits of deep sleep. Dr. Escobar is passionate about studying neuroscience; thus, he has taken part in several scientific research. As a member of three internationally-recognized sleep societies and associations, as well as having an extensive career in studying Sleep and Epilepsy, Dr. Escobar hopes to draw on his experiences to share practical knowledge with his readers. He believes that anyone can enjoy the benefits of good sleeping patterns, and his books blend simple advice with scientific insights to provide readers with the tools they need to take charge of their sleep and improve their health. Find him on:

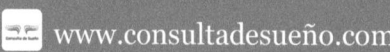 www.consultadesueño.com   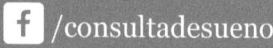 /consultadesueno

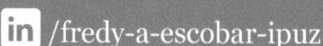 /fredy-a-escobar-ipuz   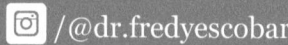 /@dr.fredyescobar

www.ingramcontent.com/pod-product-compliance
Lightning Source LLC
Chambersburg PA
CBHW040225220526
45473CB00001B/127